Slow C

Effortless Collections Of Slow Cooker Recipes For Beginners

(The Easy And Delicious Slow Cooker Recipes)

Mario Dixon

Table Of Contents

Mustard Beef 1

Beef Masala 2

Beef Sauté With Endives 4

Sweet Beef 5

Thyme Beef 7

Hot Beef 9

Beef Chops With Sprouts 10

Beef Ragout With Beans 11

Braised Beef 12

Coconut Beef 13

Beef Roast 14

Lunch Beef 15

Braised Beef Strips 16

Beef Dip 17

Beef And Sauerkraut Bowl 18

Easy Meatball Crock Pot 19

Beef & Broccoli 21

Chili Colorado 22

Mississippi Roast 23

Beef Chimichangas 25

Artichoke Pepper Beef 27

Italian Beef Roast 28

Olive Feta Beef 29

Olive Artichokes Beef 30

Sriracha Beef 32

Garlic Tomatoes Chuck Roast 33

Stuffed Bell Peppers 34

Gingerbread Pudding Cake 35

Healthy Blueberry Cobbler 38

Easy Peach Cobbler 39

Peach Compote 40

Cinnamon Apples 41

Choco Rice Pudding 42

Chocolate Fudge 43

Chocolate Brownies 45

Tasty Cherry Cobbler 46

Pineapple Cherry Dump Cake 48

Otto 49

Seafood Jambalaya 51

Spicy Pork And Butternut Squash Ragu 53

Baja Pork Tacos 56

Mexican Style Meat 58

Spicy Beef Curry 61

Beef Burritos With Green Chiles 65

Shredded Beef Lettuce Cups 68

Fajitas 71

Pot Roast With Potatoes 73

Texas-Style Baked Beans 77

Slow Cooker Bolognese 80

Layered Brisket Dinner With Tangy Mustard Sauce 84

Meatball Cabbage Rolls 88

Pulled Pork With Caramelized Onions 91

Teriyaki Pork Roast 95

Slow-Cooker Sausage & Apple Stuffing 97

Velvety Beef Steak 99

Chili Beef Roast 101

Tender Mexican Brisket 103

Beef With Tangy Horseradish Sauce 105

Sweet Potato And Pork Chops 106

North Carolina Pork Roast 109

Cranberry Pork Roast 111

Pork With Peach And Cherry Salsa 113

Cuban Orange Pork 117

Fresh Lemon Beef Goulash 120

Tuscan-Style Pork And Beans 123

Beef Picadillo 126

Pork And Potato Casserole 129

Basil Pork Chops With Grape Tomatoes 132

Chinese Ginger And Beef 135

Lean Meatloaf 138

Raspberry & Coconut Cake 141

Chocolate Cheesecake 143

Crème Brule 145

Peanut Butter & Chocolate Cake.. 146

Keto Coconut Hot Chocolate... 148

Ambrosia... 149

Dark Chocolate And Peppermint Pots................................... 152

Creamy Vanilla Custard 154

Coconut, Chocolate, And Almond Truffle Bake 155

Peanut Butter, Chocolate, And Pecan Cupcakes 157

Vanilla And Strawberry Cheesecake..................................... 160

Coffee Creams With Toasted Seed Crumble Topping... 162

Fresh Lemon Cheesecake.. 164

Apple, Avocado And Mango Bowls 166

Ricotta Cream.. 167

Tomato Jam... 169

Green Tea Pudding 170

Sweet Fresh Lemon Mix 171

Coconut Jam 172

Banana Bread 173

Bread And Berries Pudding 175

Candied Lemon 177

Tapioca And Chia Pudding 178

Mustard Beef

Ingredients:

- 2 cup of water
- 2 tablespoons mustard
- 2 tablespoon coconut oil
- 2 -pound beef sirloin, chopped
- 2 tablespoon capers, drained

Directions

1. Mix meat with mustard and leave for 25 minutes to marinate.
2. Then melt the coconut oil in the skillet.
3. Add meat and roast it for 5 minute per side on high heat.
4. After this, transfer the meat in the slow cooker.

5. Add water and capers.
6. Cook the meal on Low for 8 hours.

Beef Masala

Ingredients:
- 2 tablespoons fresh lemon juice
- 2 teaspoon ground paprika
- 1 cup of coconut milk
- 2 teaspoon dried mint
- 2 -pound beef sirloin, sliced
- 2 teaspoon g masala

Directions

1. In the bowl mix coconut milk with dried mint, ground paprika, fresh lemon juice, and g masala.

2. Then add beef sirloin and mix the mixture.
3. Leave it for at least 25 minutes to marinate.
4. Then transfer the mixture in the slow cooker.
5. Cook it on Low for 10 hours.

Beef Sauté With Endives

Ingredients:
- 2 fresh onion, sliced - 2 cup of water
- 1 cup tomato juice
- 2 -pound beef sirloin, chopped
- oz. endives, roughly chopped
- 2 teaspoon peppercorns
- 2 fresh carrot, diced

Directions
1. Mix beef with fresh onion, fresh carrot, and peppercorns.
2. Place the mixture in the slow cooker.
3. Add water and tomato juice.
4. Then close the lid and cook it on High for 6 hours.
5. After this, add endives and cook the meal for 4 hours on Low.

Sweet Beef

Ingredients:
- 2 tablespoons fresh lemon juice
- 2 teaspoon dried oregano
- 2 cup of water
- 2 -pound beef roast, sliced
- 2 tablespoon maple syrup

Directions
1. Mix water with maple syrup, fresh lemon juice, and dried oregano.
2. Then pour the liquid in the slow cooker.
3. Add beef roast and close the lid.
4. Cook the meal on High for 6 hours.

Thyme Beef

Ingredients:
- 2 tablespoon olive oil
- 1 cup of water
- 2 teaspoon salt
- oz. beef sirloin, chopped
- 2 tablespoon dried thyme

Directions
1. Preheat the skillet well.
2. Then mix beef with dried thyme and olive oil.
3. Put the meat in the hot skillet and roast for 5 minutes per side on high heat.
4. Then transfer the meat in the slow cooker.
5. Add salt and water.
6. Cook the meal on High for 6 hours.

Hot Beef

Ingredients:
- 2 tablespoons hot sauce
- 2 tablespoon olive oil - 1 cup of water
  2 -pound beef sirloin, chopped

Directions

1. In the shallow bowl mix hot sauce with olive oil.
2. Then mix beef sirloin with hot sauce mixture and leave for 25 minutes to marinate.
3. Put the marinated beef in the slow cooker.
4. Add water and close the lid.
5. Cook the meal on Low for 8 hours.

Beef Chops With Sprouts

Ingredients:
- 2 teaspoon chili powder
- 2 teaspoon salt
- 2 -pound beef loin - 1 cup bean sprouts
- 2 cup of water - 2 tablespoon tomato paste

Directions

1. Cut the beef loin into 6 beef chops and sprinkle the beef chops with chili powder and salt.
2. Then place them in the slow cooker.
3. Add water and tomato paste.
4. Cook the meat on low for 8 hours.
5. Then transfer the cooked beef chops in the plates, sprinkle with tomato gravy from the slow cooker, and top with bean sprouts.

Beef Ragout With Beans

Ingredients:
- 2 -pound beef stew meat, chopped
- 2 teaspoon ground black pepper
- 2 cups of water 2 tablespoon tomato paste
- 2 cup mug beans, canned - 2 fresh carrot, grated

Directions
1. Pour water in the slow cooker.
2. Add meat, ground black pepper, and carrot.
3. Cook the mixture on High for 4 hours.
4. Then add tomato paste and mug beans.
5. Stir the meal and cook it on high for 2 hour more.

Braised Beef

Ingredients:

- 2 teaspoon salt
- 2 tablespoon dried basil
- 2 cups of water
- oz. beef tenderloin, chopped
- 2 garlic clove, peeled
- 2 teaspoon peppercorn

Directions

1. Put all ingredients from the list above in the slow cooker.
2. Gently stir the mixture and close the lid.
3. Cook the beef on low for 10 hours.

Coconut Beef

Ingredients:

- 2 -pound beef tenderloin, chopped
- 2 teaspoon avocado oil
- 2 teaspoon dried rosemary
- 2 teaspoon garlic powder
- 2 cup baby spinach, chopped
- 2 cup of coconut milk

Directions

1. Roast meat in the avocado oil for 5 minute per side on high heat.
2. Ten transfer the meat in the slow cooker.
3. Add garlic powder, dried rosemary, coconut milk, and baby spinach.
4. Close the lid and cook the meal on Low for 8 hours.

Beef Roast

Ingredients:
- 2 teaspoon chili powder
- 2 teaspoon olive oil
- 2 teaspoon fresh lemon juice
- 1 cup of water
- 2 -pound beef chuck roast
- 2 tablespoon ketchup
- 2 tablespoon mayonnaise

Directions
1. In the bowl mix ketchup, mayonnaise, chili powder, olive oil, and fresh lemon juice.
2. Then sprinkle the beef chuck roast with ketchup mixture.
3. Pour the water in the slow cooker.
4. Add beef chuck roast and close the lid.
5. Cook the meat on High for 6 hours.

Lunch Beef

Ingredients:

- 2 teaspoon hot sauce
- 1 cup okra, chopped
- 2 cup of water
- oz. beef loin, chopped 1 white fresh onion, sliced
- 2 teaspoon brown sugar
- 2 teaspoon chili powder

Directions

1. Mix the beef loin with hot sauce, chili powder, and brown sugar.
2. Transfer the meat in the slow cooker.
3. Add water, okra, and onion.
4. Cook the meal on Low for 8 hours.

Braised Beef Strips

Ingredients:
- 2 tablespoon coconut oil
- 2 teaspoon salt
- 2 teaspoon white pepper
- oz. beef loin, cut into strips
- 1 cup mushroom, sliced
- 2 fresh onion, sliced
- 2 cup of water

Directions
1. Melt the coconut oil in the skillet.
2. Add mushrooms and roast them for 6 minutes on medium heat.
3. Then transfer the mushrooms in the slow cooker.
4. Add all remaining ingredients and close the lid.
5. Cook the meal on High for 6 hours

Beef Dip

Ingredients:

- 1 cup Cheddar cheese, shredded
- 2 teaspoon garlic powder
- oz. dried beef, chopped
- 1 cup of water 1 cup heavy cream
- 2 fresh onion, diced
- 2 teaspoon cream cheese

Directions

1. Put all ingredients in the slow cooker.
2. Gently stir the ingredients and close the lid.
3. Cook the dip on Low for 25 hours.

Beef And Sauerkraut Bowl

Ingredients:
- 1/2 cup apple cider vinegar
- 2 cup of water
- 2 cup sauerkraut
- 2 -pound corned beef, chopped

Directions
1. Pour water and apple cider vinegar in the slow cooker.
2. Add corned beef and cook it on High for 6 hours.
3. Then chop the meat roughly and put in the serving bowls.
4. Top the meat with sauerkraut.

Easy Meatball Crock Pot

Ingredients:

- For the meatballs:
- 2 lb. ground beef
- Fresh handful fresh parsley, diced
- For the cauliflower:
- Sea salt
- 2 tablespoons butter or ghee
- 1 large head cauliflower, florets
- Pepper
- 2 tablespoon tomato paste
- 2 cup bone broth - Sea salt and pepper
- 1 teaspoon paprika
- 1 tablespoon cumin

Directions:

1. Mix the meat, pepper, salt, paprika, and cumin in a bowl.
2. Form meatballs, then put it inside the slow cooker.

3. Mix the paste and the broth in a bowl and pour over the meatballs.
4. Cook on high, 2 hours.
5. Steam the cauliflower florets until well cooked.
6. Remove the water, then put salt, butter, plus pepper.
7. Blend the batter using an immersion blender until smooth.
8. Mash the cauliflower onto a serving plate, top with meatballs, and enough amount of sauce on top.
9. Garnish with parsley and enjoy.

Beef & Broccoli

Ingredients:

- 4 garlic cloves, minced
- 2 tsp grated ginger - 4 tbsp sweetener
- 2 cup beef broth
- 1/2 cup liquid amigos
- 2 lbs. flank steak, chunks
- 2 tsp sesame seeds,
- 2 red bell pepper, sliced - 2 broccoli, florets
- 1 tsp salt - 1/2 tsp red pepper flakes

Directions:

1. Set the slow cooker on low, put the steak, salt, pepper, garlic, sweetener, beef broth, and coconut aminos.
2. Cook within 5 to 7 hours.
3. Mix the steak, then put in the red pepper plus the broccoli.
4. Cook within 2 hour, then toss the batter.

5. Serve with sesame seeds.

Chili Colorado

Ingredients:

- 2 teaspoon salt - 0.6 teaspoons chili powder
- 2 onion - 44 .6 ounces tomatoes, canned
- 2 teaspoon ground cumin
- 2 teaspoon pepper
- 2.6 pounds beef - 4 cloves garlic
- 28 ounces green chilies, canned

Directions:
1. Put the meat in the cooker.
2. Add the garlic and onion.
3. Add the tomatoes and chilies.

4. Add the seasonings.
5. Low cook for 25 hours. Serve.

Mississippi Roast

Ingredients:
- 4 tablespoons olive oil
- 2 yellow onion - 2 cup au jus
- 6 pepperoncini
- 2 pounds roast beef
- 2 pack dressing mix, ranch
- 0.6 cups butter, salted

Directions:

1. Sear the roast.
2. Cover with chopped onion.
3. Pour in au jus.
4. Sprinkle ranch mix.
5. Evenly disperse the butter.
6. Evenly place pepperoncini.

7. Low cook for 8 hours.

Beef Chimichangas

Ingredients:

- 4 garlic cloves
- 2 6 flour tortillas
- Toppings: - Refried beans
- Sour cream
- Guacamole
- Lettuce - Cheese
- Salsa
- 4 pounds beef, boneless
- 25 ounces green chilies and tomatoes, canned
- 4 ounces garlic
- 4 tablespoons seasoning, taco

Directions:

1. Prepare the meat. Add it to the cooker after applying seasoning.
2. Add chilies and tomatoes. Toss in garlic.
3. Low cook for 7 hours.
4. Shred the beef.
5. Once removed, add it and all desired toppings to tortillas.
6. Fry folded tortillas. Serve.

Artichoke Pepper Beef

Ingredients:

- 2 cups marinara sauce
- 2 tsp dried basil
- 2 tsp dried oregano
- 7 oz roasted red peppers, drained and sliced
- 2 lbs stew beef, cut into 2 -inch cubes
- 7 oz artichoke hearts, drained
- 2 fresh onion, diced

Directions:

1. Add all ingredients into the cooking pot and stir well.
2. Cover instant pot aura with lid.
3. Select slow cook mode and cook on LOW for 6 hours.
4. Stir well and serve.

Italian Beef Roast

Ingredients:

- 1/2 cup sun-dried tomatoes, chopped
- 8 garlic cloves, chopped
- 1/2 cup fresh parsley, chopped
- 1/2 cup olives, chopped –
- 1 cup chicken stock
- 2 lbs chuck roast, boneless
- 2 tbsp balsamic vinegar
- 2 tsp herb de Provence

Directions:

1. Add all ingredients into the cooking pot and stir well.
2. Cover instant pot aura with lid.
3. Select slow cook mode and cook on LOW for 6 hours.
4. Remove meat from pot and shred using a fork.
5. Serve and enjoy.

Olive Feta Beef

Ingredients:

45 oz can tomato, diced

1 cup feta cheese, crumbled

1/2 tsp pepper

7 tsp salt

2 lbs beef stew meat, cut into half-inch pieces

2 cup olives, pitted and cut in half

Directions:

1. Add all ingredients into the cooking pot and stir well.
2. Cover instant pot aura with lid.
3. Select slow cook mode and cook on HIGH for 6 hours.
4. Serve and enjoy.

Olive Artichokes Beef

Ingredients:
- 2 bay leaf
- 1 tsp ground cumin
- 2 tsp dried basil
- 2 tsp dried parsley
- 4 garlic cloves, chopped
- 2 fresh onion, diced
- 2 4 oz can artichoke hearts, drained and halved
- 2 tbsp olive oil
- 2 lbs stew beef, cut into 2 -inch cubes
- 2 tsp dried oregano
- 1 cup olives, pitted and chopped
- 2 4 oz can tomato, diced
- 30 oz can tomato sauce
- 4 2 oz chicken stock

Directions:

1. Add the meat into the cooking pot then mix together the remaining ingredients and pour over the meat.
2. Cover instant pot aura with lid.
3. Select slow cook mode and cook on LOW for 8 hours.
4. Stir well and serve.

Sriracha Beef

Ingredients:
- 2 cup beef broth
- 1 medium fresh onion, sliced
- 2 cups bell pepper, chopped
- 2 tsp black pepper
- 2 tsp salt
- 2 lbs beef chuck, sliced
- 2 tbsp sriracha sauce
- 1/2 cup parsley, chopped
- 2 tsp garlic powder

Directions:
1. Add the meat into the cooking pot then mix together the remaining ingredients and pour over the meat.
2. Cover instant pot aura with lid.
3. Select slow cook mode and cook on HIGH for 4 hours.
4. Stir well and serve.

Garlic Tomatoes Chuck Roast

Ingredients:

- 26 garlic cloves, peeled
- 1/2 cup olives, sliced
- 2 tsp dried Italian seasoning, crushed
- 2 tbsp balsamic vinegar
- 2 lbs beef chuck roast
- 1 cup beef broth
- 1/2 cup sun-dried tomatoes, chopped

Directions:

1. Add the meat into the cooking pot then mix together the remaining ingredients except for couscous and pour over the meat.
2. Cover instant pot aura with lid. Select slow cook mode and cook on LOW for 8 hours.

3. Remove meat from pot and shred using a fork.
4. Return shredded meat to the pot and stir well.

Stuffed Bell Peppers

Ingredients:

1 lb ground breakfast sausage

4 bell pepper, cut top and clean

2 /8 tsp black pepper

1/2 tsp salt

6 large fresh eggs

4 oz green chilies, chopped

4 oz jack cheese, shredded

Directions:

1. Brown sausage in a pan over medium heat.
2. Drain excess grease.

3. Pour 1 cup water in the cooking pot. In a bowl, whisk eggs until smooth.
4. Stir green chilies, cheese, black pepper, and salt in eggs.
5. Spoon egg mixture and brown sausage into each bell pepper.
6. Place stuffed bell pepper in the cooking pot.
7. Cover instant pot aura with lid.
8. Select slow cook mode and cook on LOW for 4 hours.

Gingerbread Pudding Cake

Ingredients:

- 2 cup of water
- 1 cup molasses
- 2 tsp vanilla
- 1/2 cup sugar
- 1/2 cup butter, softened

- 1/2 tsp salt
- 2 egg
- 2 1/2 cups whole wheat flour
- 2 /8 tsp ground nutmeg
- 1 tsp ground ginger
- 1 tsp ground cinnamon
- 1/3 tsp baking soda

Directions:
1. In a bowl, beat sugar and butter until combined.
2. Add egg and beat until combined.
3. Add water, molasses, and vanilla and beat until well combined.
4. Add flour, nutmeg, ginger, cinnamon, baking soda, and salt and stir until combined.
5. Pour batter into the cooking pot.
6. Cover instant pot aura with lid.
7. Select slow cook mode and cook on HIGH for 4 hours.
8. Serve with vanilla ice-cream.

Healthy Blueberry Cobbler

Ingredients:

- 2 tsp cinnamon
- 2 tbsp cornstarch
- 4 1 tsp baking powder
- 2 1/2 cups sugar
- 2 tsp salt
- 2 1/2 cups all-purpose flour
- 4 cups blueberries
- 8 tbsp butter, melted

Directions:

1. Add blueberries into the cooking pot.
2. Mix together flour, cinnamon, cornstarch, baking powder, sugar, and salt and sprinkle over blueberries evenly.

3. Pour melted butter over flour mixture evenly.
4. Cover instant pot aura with lid.
5. Select slow cook mode and cook on LOW for 4 hours.

Easy Peach Cobbler

Ingredients:

- 2 box cake mix
- 45 oz can sliced peaches in syrup
- 1 cup butter, cut into pieces

Directions:

1. Add sliced peaches with syrup into the cooking pot.
2. Sprinkle cake mix on top of sliced peaches.
3. Spread butter pieces on top of the cake mix.
4. Cover instant pot aura with lid.

5. Select slow cook mode and cook on HIGH for 4 hours.
6. Serve with vanilla ice-cream.

Peach Compote

Ingredients:

- 1/2 cup butter, cut into pieces
- 1 cup brown sugar
- 1 cup sugar
- 8 ripe peaches, peeled & sliced
- 2 tsp vanilla
- 2 tsp cinnamon

Directions:

1. Add peaches, vanilla, cinnamon, brown sugar, and sugar into the cooking pot and stir well.

2. Spread butter pieces on top of the peach mixture.
3. Cover instant pot aura with lid.
4. Select slow cook mode and cook on LOW for 2 hours.
5. Serve with vanilla ice-cream.

Cinnamon Apples

Ingredients:

- 2 tbsp cornstarch
- 2 tbsp maple syrup
- 1/2 cup apple cider
- 6 apples, peeled and sliced
- 2 1/2 tsp ground cinnamon

Directions:

1. In a bowl, mix together apple cider, cinnamon, cornstarch, maple syrup, and 1/2 cup water.

2. Add apples into the cooking pot the pour apple cider mixture over apples.
3. Cover instant pot aura with lid.
4. Select slow cook mode and cook on LOW for 2 hours.
5. Stir after 2 hour.
6. Stir well and serve.

Choco Rice Pudding

Ingredients:

- 2 4 oz coconut milk
- 7 oz can evaporate milk
- 4 cups of water
- 1 cup cocoa powder
- 2 cups sticky rice, rinsed & drained
- 1 cup chocolate chips
- 1 cup brown sugar

Directions:

1. Add rice, water, and cocoa powder into the cooking pot and stir well.
2. Cover instant pot aura with lid.
3. Select slow cook mode and cook on HIGH for 2 hours.
4. Add remaining ingredients and stir everything well, cover, and cook for 45 minutes more.
5. Serve and enjoy.

Chocolate Fudge

Ingredients:

- 2 tbsp butter
- 2 tsp vanilla
- 4 cups chocolate chips

Directions:

1. Add all ingredients into the cooking pot and stir well.

2. Select slow cook mode and cook on LOW for 2 hour.
3. Stir after every 30 minutes.
4. Once done, pour into the greased tin.
5. Place in the fridge for 2 hours or until set.
6. Cut into pieces and serve

Chocolate Brownies

Ingredients:

- 1/2 cup unsweetened cocoa powder
- 1/2 cup brown sugar
- 2 1/2 cup sugar
- 1 tsp salt
- 4 fresh eggs
- 2 cup butter, melted
- 2 cup peanut butter chips
- 2 tsp vanilla
- 1/2 cup all-purpose flour

Directions:

1. Line instant pot aura cooking pot with parchment paper.
2. In a mixing bowl, beat butter, sugar, brown sugar, cocoa powder, flour,

fresh eggs, vanilla, and salt until smooth.
3. Add peanut butter chips to the batter and fold well.
4. Pour batter into the cooking pot.
5. Cover instant pot aura with lid.
6. Select slow cook mode and cook on LOW for 4 hours.
7. Slice and serve.

Tasty Cherry Cobbler

Ingredients:

- 2 box cake mix
- 45 oz can cherry pie filling 1
- cup butter, cut into pieces

Directions:

1. Add cherry pie filling into the cooking pot, then sprinkle cake mix over cherry pie filling evenly.
2. Spread butter pieces on top of the cake mix.
3. Cover instant pot aura with lid.
4. Select slow cook mode and cook on HIGH for 2 hours.
5. Serve and enjoy.

Pineapple Cherry Dump Cake

Ingredients:

- 4 stick butter, cubed
- 2 box cake mix
- 30 oz can cherry pie filling
- 30 oz can pineapple, crushed
- 1/3 cup pecans, chopped

Directions:

1. Add cherry pie filling and crushed pineapple into the cooking pot and stir well.
2. Sprinkle cake mix over cherry pie filling mixture evenly.
3. Spread butter pieces and pecans on top of cake mix.
4. Cover instant pot aura with lid.

5. Select slow cook mode and cook on HIGH for 4 hours.
6. Serve and enjoy.

Otto

Ingredients:

- 4 cups low sodium vegetable broth
- 1/2 cup dry white wine
- 2 /8 tsp ground black pepper
- 1 lb salmon fillet, cubed
- 4 Tbsp unsalted butter
- 4 oz Arborio rice
- 2 Tbsp minced onion

Instructions:

1. Place a skillet over medium high flame and melt the butter.

2. Add the minced onion and sauté until translucent, then scrape mixture into the slow cooker.

3. Pour the Arborio rice into the slow cooker, followed by the broth, wine, and black pepper.

4. Cover and cook for 4 hours on low, stirring once halfway into the cooking time.

5. Add the salmon and stir to distribute.

6. Cover and cook for 45 minutes on high or until salmon is cooked through and rice is puffed and tender. Serve warm.

Seafood Jambalaya

Ingredients:

- 1/2 tsp hot pepper sauce
- 1/2 tsp cayenne pepper
- 1/2 tsp cracked black pepper
- 1/2 tsp sea salt
- 1/2 tsp dried thyme
- 1/2 tsp dried oregano
- 1 bay leaf
- 1/2 cup chopped fresh parsley
- 1 lb fresh shrimp, shelled and deveined
- 1 lb fresh bay scallops
- 4 cups cooked long grain brown rice
- Juice and zest of 1 fresh lemon
- A dash of xylitol
- 2 4 oz diced tomatoes, not drained
- 2 fresh yellow fresh onion, chopped

- 2 celery ribs, sliced thinly
- 8 oz crushed tomatoes
- 2 bell pepper, seeded and chopped
- 4 garlic cloves, minced
- 1 tsp dried oregano
- 1 tsp sweet paprika

Instructions:

1. Mix together the fresh onion, tomatoes, celery, peppers, bay leaf, garlic, fresh lemon zest, thyme, paprika, oregano, hot sauce, peppers, sea salt, and xylitol.

2. Cover and cook for 4 hours on high or for 6 hours on low.

3. Set heat to high, then stir in the scallops and shrimp.

4. Cover and cook again for 30 minutes, or until the seafood is cooked through.

5. Stir in the parsley and fresh lemon juice, then spoon on top of the cooked brown rice and serve.

Spicy Pork And Butternut Squash Ragu

Ingredients:

- Shaved parmesan cheese to serve
- 6 oz frozen cooked winter squash, thawed
- 2 fresh sweet red pepper, cut into 1 inch dice
- 2 /8 tsp garlic powder
- 2 tsp crushed red pepper flakes

- Hot cooked pasta or zucchini noodles or any other low carb pasta, to serve
- 2 canstewed tomatoes, with its liquid
- 2 medium sweet fresh onion, cut into 1 inch dice
- 2 lb country style pork ribs, boneless
- Freshly ground black pepper to taste
- Salt to taste
- Pepper to taste

Instructions:

1. Add stewed tomatoes, fresh onion, red pepper, squash and red pepper flakes into the slow cooker.
2. Stir until well combined.

3. Sprinkle salt, pepper and garlic powder all over the pork and place over the onion mixture in the slow cooker.
4. Cover and cook for 6 -6 hours or for 4 - 4 hours on high or until pork is cooked well and coming off the bones.
5. Uncover and mix well.
6. Serve over pasta, garnished with shaved parmesan cheese if using.

Baja Pork Tacos

Ingredients:

- 7 corn tortillas warmed according to the instructions on the package
- ¾ cup shredded, part-skim mozzarella cheese
- 4 cans chopped green chilies
- 4 tsp ground cumin
- 4 cups shredded lettuce
- 4 lb pork sirloin roast, halved
- 2 Tbsp reduced sodium taco seasoning

Instructions:

1. Place pork roast in the slow cooker.
2. Add chilies, cumin and taco seasoning into a bowl and spread all over the pork.
3. Cover and cook for 10 hours on low or 4 -4 hours on high or until cooked through.
4. Remove pork with a slotted spoon and place on your cutting board.
5. When cool enough to handle, shred the meat with a pair of forks.
6. Carefully remove the fat floating on the top of the cooked liquid from the slow cooker.
7. Discard the fat.
8. Add shredded meat back into the slow cooker.
9. Mix well.
10. Cook for 1 to 5 until well heated.
11. Spread tortillas on your countertop.

12. Place lettuce and cheese on the tortillas.
13. Top with shredded pork and serve.

Mexican Style Meat

Ingredients:

- 1 bottleot pepper sauce
- 1 tsp salt or to taste
- 2 Tbsp olive oil
- 1 - ¾ cup diced green chili pepper
- 1 tsp ground cayenne pepper
- 1 tsp garlic powder
- Tacos or burritos, to serve
- 2 lb chuck roast, trimmed of excess fat
- 1 tsp ground black pepper
- 2 medium fresh onion, chopped
- 1 tsp chili powder

Instructions:

1. Place a skillet over medium-high heat. Add oil and let it heat. Sprinkle salt and pepper all over the roast and place in the skillet.
2. Cook until brown all over. Turn off the heat.
3. Remove the roast from the skillet and place in the slow cooker.
4. Scatter onions over the roast.
5. Also spread the chili peppers over the onions.
6. Sprinkle cayenne pepper, chili powder, garlic powder and hot sauce.
7. Pour water to cover at least 1/2 of the roast.
8. Cover and cook for 6 hours on High after which cook for 2-4 hours on low or until the meat falls off the bones.

9. Remove meat with a slotted spoon and place on your cutting board.
10. When cool enough to handle, shred the meat with a pair of forks.
11. Remove 2 -2 cups of the cooked liquid and use in some other recipe or discard it.
12. Add the shredded meat back into the slow cooker. Mix well.

Spicy Beef Curry

Ingredients:
- 1 tsp ground coriander
- 1 tsp salt
- 1 tsp ground cumin
- 1 tsp turmeric
- 4 oz fat free Greek yogurt
- 2 lb lean, braising / casserole steak, chopped into fresh chunks

For curry:
- 2 dried whole chilies
- 2 cloves garlic, peeled, minced
- 2 Tbsp tomato paste
- 1 can chopped tomatoes
- A handful fresh cilantro, chopped, to garnish
- 6 sprays light cooking oil spray
- 2 Tbsp ground coriander

- 4 pods cardamom
- ¾ Tbsp ground cumin
- 2 tsp garam masala
- 1 tsp turmeric
- Freshly ground black pepper to taste
- 2 fresh fresh green chili, finely chopped
- 2 inch fresh ginger, peeled, minced
- 2 cup beef stock or 2 cup water mixed with 2 beef stock cube or 2 tsp beef bouillon
- Juice of 1 fresh lemon
- 2 medium fresh onion, chopped

Serving options:
- Cucumber raita
- Cooked brown rice or white rice
- Cauliflower rice

Instructions:

1. For beef: Add yogurt, coriander, salt, cumin and turmeric into a bowl and mix until well combined.
2. Add beef and mix well using your hands.
3. Rub it well onto the beef.
4. Cover the bowl with cling wrap and chill for 2-8 hours.
5. Place a pan over high heat.
6. Spray 6 sprays of cooking spray.
7. Remove beef from the refrigerator and place in the pan. Cook until brown.
8. Drain the cooked liquid from the pan.
9. Add onion and sauté until translucent.
10. Stir in cumin, turmeric, black pepper, chopped chilies, ginger, garlic, coriander, cardamom, garam masala and whole chilies. Sauté until fragrant.

11. Add tomato paste, chopped tomatoes, stock and fresh lemon juice and mix well.
12. Cover and cook for 5 to 7 hours on low or for 4 to 4 hours on high.
13. Add salt and pepper to taste.
i. Serve over your preferred rice and with some cucumber raita if desired.

Beef Burritos With Green Chiles

Ingredients:

- 2 canswhole green chilies, drained, coarsely chopped
- 8 whole wheat tortillas warmed according to the instructions on the package
- 1 tsp salt

- 1 tsp cayenne pepper
- 1 can (from a 28 oz can) diced tomatoes
- 2 medium fresh onion, chopped
- 2 clove garlic, peeled, minced
- 2 tsp ground cumin
- 2 lb beef chuck roast

Optional toppings: *Use any*
- 1 cup sour cream
- 1/2 cup sliced ripe olives
- Or any other toppings of your choice
- 1 cup salsa
- 1 cup shredded cheddar cheese

Instructions:

1. Add salt, garlic, cayenne pepper and cumin into a bowl and stir.
2. Rub this mixture well onto the roast.
3. Place roast in the slow cooker.
4. Stir in the tomatoes, onion and chili.
5. Cover and cook for 8 to 8 hours or until cooked through.
6. Remove beef with a slotted spoon and place on your cutting board.
7. When cool enough to handle, shred the meat with a pair of forks.
8. Drain off the excess liquid from the cooking pot (do not discard the vegetables).
9. Add beef into the pot. Mix well.
10. Heat thoroughly.
11. Spread the tortillas on your countertop.
12. Divide the meat and vegetables over the tortillas.
13. Place the toppings if using and serve.

Shredded Beef Lettuce Cups

Ingredients:
- 2 Tbsp water
- 2 Tbsp brown sugar
- 2 clove garlic, peeled, minced
- 4 Tbsp cornstarch
- 7 Bibb or Boston lettuce leaves
- 1 can crushed pineapple, unsweetened, with its liquid
- 2 green fresh onion, thinly sliced, to garnish
- 2 lb beef chuck roast
- 2 medium sweet pepper, chopped
- 4 fresh carrots, peeled, chopped
- 2 fresh fresh onion, chopped

- 1/2 cup low sodium soy sauce
- 2 Tbsp white vinegar
- 1/2 tsp pepper

Instructions:

1. Add fresh carrot, fresh onion, pepper and chuck roast into the slow cooker.
2. Add soy sauce, white vinegar, pepper, water, brown sugar and garlic into a bowl and stir.
3. Pour all over the vegetables and roast in the slow cooker.
4. Cover and cook for 6 to 8 hours or until roast is cooked through.
5. Remove roast with a slotted spoon and place on your cutting board.
6. When cool enough to handle, shred the meat with a pair of forks.
7. Carefully remove any fat that is floating on top from the slow cooker.
8. Discard the fat. Pour the liquid remaining in the pot into a saucepan.

9. Place saucepan over medium heat.
10. Mix together cornstarch and a little water in a bowl and pour into the saucepan.
11. Whisk constantly until the mixture thickens.
12. Turn off the heat and pour the thickened sauce into the slow cooker.
13. Add the shredded meat into the slow cooker and stir until well coated.
14. Heat thoroughly.
i. Place the lettuce cups on a serving platter. Divide the meat and vegetable mixture into the lettuce cups.
ii. Garnish with green onions and serve.

Fajitas

Ingredients:
- 2 medium fresh onion, thinly sliced
- 2 Tbsp canola oil
- 2 fresh clove garlic, peeled, minced
- 2 medium bell pepper, cut into thin strips
- 4 mini whole wheat tortillas
- ¾ lb beef top sirloin steak, cut into thin strips
- 2 Tbsp fresh lemon juice
- ¾ tsp ground cumin
- 1/2 tsp chili powder
- 1 tsp seasoned salt
- 1/2 tsp crushed red pepper flakes

Optional toppings:
- 2 jalapeño, deseed if desired, thinly sliced
- A handful fresh cilantro, chopped

- 2 fresh avocado, peeled, pitted, sliced
- 1 cup shredded cheddar cheese

Instructions:
1. Place a skillet over medium heat.
2. Add oil and heat. When the oil is heated, add steak and cook until brown all over.
3. Turn off the heat.
4. Transfer the steak with all the cooked liquid into the slow cooker.
5. Add garlic, fresh lemon juice, chili powder, cumin, red pepper flakes and salt and mix well.
6. Cover and cook for 2 hours on high or until meat is nearly cooked.
7. Stir in the onion and red pepper.
8. Cover and continue cooking until the meat is well cooked.
9. Heat the tortillas following the instructions on the package.

10. Place tortillas on a serving platter.
11. Divide the beef and vegetables along the diameter of the tortillas.
12. Place the optional toppings if desired and serve.

Pot Roast With Potatoes

Ingredients:
- 2 tsp garlic, minced
- 2 medium fresh onion, sliced
- 2 Tbsp Worcestershire sauce
- 1 Tbsp cornstarch mixed with 2 Tbsp water
- 1 Tbsp salt
- 1 tsp dried thyme or 2 Tbsp fresh thyme, chopped (optional)

- 2 tsp pepper powder or to taste
- 4 lb extra- lean eye of round beef roast
- 2 lb potatoes, cubed
- 1 lb carrots, peeled, cubed

Instructions:

1. Spread the cornstarch mixture on the bottom of the slow cooker.

2. Place fresh onion, garlic, carrot and potatoes in the pot.

3. Sprinkle salt, thyme and pepper powder.

4. Mix well and transfer into the pot.

5. Sprinkle salt and pepper over the beef and place it in the pot, over the vegetables.

6. Drizzle Worcestershire sauce on top.

7. Cover and cook for 8 to 25 hours on low or 4 to 6 hours on high.

8. Remove the beef with a slotted spoon and place on your cutting board.

9. When cool enough to handle, slice the beef against the grain.

10. If the gravy in the pot is watery, transfer into a pan.

11. Place pan over medium heat and boil until it thickens as per your liking.

12. Pour sauce over the beef slices and serve.

Texas-Style Baked Beans

Ingredients:
- 1 cup barbeque sauce
- 1 Tbsp garlic powder
- 4 Tbsp hot sauce of your choice, or to taste
- 4 2 oz canned baked beans with pork
- 1 fresh Vidalia fresh onion, peeled, chopped
- 1/2 cup brown sugar
- 1 Tbsp chili powder
- 1 lb ground beef
- 2 oz canned chopped green chili peppers

Instructions:

1. Place a skillet over medium heat.
2. Add beef and cook until it is not pink anymore.
3. Drain fat remaining in the pan.
4. Break it simultaneously as it cooks.
5. Transfer the beef into the slow cooker.
6. Add baked beans, fresh onion, green chili, garlic powder, brown sugar, hot sauce, chili sauce and barbeque sauce.
7. Cover and cook for 2 hours on high or for 4 – 6 hours on low.

Slow Cooker Bolognese

Ingredients:
- 2 Tbsp white wine
- 2 bay leaves
- 2 Tbsp fresh parsley, chopped
- 1 Tbsp butter or olive oil
- 28 oz canned, crushed tomatoes
- Salt to taste
- Pepper to taste
- 1/2 cup half and half
- Low carb noodles of your choice to serve
- 2 oz pancetta, chopped or center cut bacon
- 2 medium white fresh onion, minced
- 2 medium fresh carrot, minced
- 2 celery stalk, minced
- 2 lb 10 6 % lean ground beef

Instructions:

1. Place a skillet over low heat.
2. Add pancetta and cook until fat is released.
3. Raise the heat to medium-low.
4. Stir in the butter, celery, onions and carrots and cook until slightly tender.
5. Raise the heat to medium- high.
6. Add beef, salt and pepper and cook until brown.
7. Drain excess fat in the pan.
8. Add in the wine and stir.
9. Cook until it is reduced to half its original quantity.
10. Turn off the heat.
11. Place tomatoes, salt, pepper and bay leaves in the slow cooker.

12. Transfer meat into the cooker. Mix well.

13. Cover and cook for 6 -6 hours on Low or 2-4 hours on high.

14. Taste and adjust the seasoning if necessary.

15. Stir in half and half and parsley.

16. Serve over low carb noodles.

Layered Brisket Dinner With Tangy Mustard Sauce

Ingredients:

- ¾ tsp Dijon style mustard
- 1/2 tsp snipped fresh thyme
- 1/2 cup light sour cream
- 1/2 tsp dried Italian seasoning, crushed

For Layered brisket

- 2 tsp olive oil
- Salt to taste
- Snipped fresh thyme
- 1 Tbsp Dijon style mustard
- 1 Tbsp balsamic vinegar

- 1 lb baby potatoes, red or yellow, halved if large
- 1 fresh fresh onion, cut into wedges
- 1/2 tsp dried Italian seasoning, crushed
- 4 lb fresh beef brisket, trimmed of fat
- 1 Tbsp Worcestershire sauce
- Pepper to taste
- 4 oz baby carrots

Instructions:

1. For tangy mustard sauce:
2. Whisk together sour cream, thyme, Italian seasoning and mustard in a bowl.
3. Cover and refrigerate until use.
4. For layered brisket: Lay the brisket in the slow cooker.

5. Add mustard, vinegar, pepper powder and Worcestershire sauce into a fresh bowl and whisk well.

6. Spread the sauce mixture over the brisket.

7. Turn the brisket and spread the sauce mixture on the other side of the brisket.

8. Take a large sheet of heavy foil.

9. Lay carrots, potato and onion over it. Pour oil over the vegetables and toss well.

10. Season with salt, pepper and Italian seasoning.

11. Seal completely and place in the slow cooker, over the brisket.

12. Cover the pot and cook for 8-10 hours on Low.

13. Remove brisket from the pot and place on your cutting board.

14. When cool enough to handle, cut into slices or shred with a pair of forks.

15. Unfold the foil packet just before serving.

16. Serve brisket slices topped with the vegetables.

17. Serve with tangy mustard sauce.

18. Garnish with thyme and serve.

Meatball Cabbage Rolls

Ingredients:

- 10 oz canned tomato sauce
- 4 oz canned, unsalted tomato sauce
- 4 Tbsp uncooked long grain rice
- 2 /8 tsp garlic powder
- 1 lb 10 0% lean ground beef, crumbled
- 2 large heads cabbage
- 2 fresh onions, chopped
- 2 Tbsp chili powder
- Salt to taste

Instructions:

1. Place a large saucepan or Dutch oven filled with water over high heat.

2. When the water begins to boil, drop the cabbages in the pot.

3. You can cook in batches if your saucepan is not large enough.

4. Cook until the leaves are coming off the head.

5. Do not overcook.

6. Pull out 7 outer leaves from each of the cabbage.

7. The inner part of the cabbage can be used in some other recipe.

8. Make a V shaped cut all along the sides of the thick vein and remove the vein.

9. Add unsalted tomato sauce, chili powder, fresh onion, rice, salt and garlic powder into a bowl and stir.

10. Add beef and mix until well combined.

11. Divide the mixture into 24 equal portions and shape into balls.

12. Spread the cooked cabbage leaves on your countertop.

13. Place a meatball on each. Fold the sides, over the meatballs to cover completely.

14. Fasten with toothpicks.

15. Place cabbage meatballs in the slow cooker.

16. Spoon the tomato sauce over the meatballs.

17. Cover and cook for 8 hours on low or until meat is cooked.

18. Serve after discarding the toothpicks.

Pulled Pork With Caramelized Onions

Ingredients:
- 2 Tbsp extra virgin olive oil
- 4 lb pork shoulder or blade roast, boneless, trimmed
- 4 Tbsp raw cane sugar
- 4 Tbsp apple cider vinegar
- 1 tsp dried oregano
- 1 tsp salt or to taste
- 1 cup chili sauce
- 2 -2 tsp chipotle chili in adobo sauce
- 4 medium onions, thinly sliced
- 2 cloves garlic, minced
- 1 tsp freshly ground pepper

Instructions:

1. Place a skillet over medium high heat.
2. Add oil and heat.
3. Add onions and cook until translucent.
4. Add sugar and cook until the onions are caramelized.
5. Stir constantly.
6. Add garlic, oregano, pepper, salt and cook until aromatic.
7. Add vinegar and simmer until almost dry.
8. Remove from heat.
9. Add chili sauce and chipotle chili and stir until well combined

10. Place pork in the slow cooker.

11. Pour the cooked sauce over the pork.

12. Cover and cook on Low for 8-10 hours.

13. The meat should be falling off the bone.

14. When done, remove pork and place on your cutting board.

15. When cool enough to handle, shred the pork using a pair of forks.

16. Add the pork back to the pot and heat thoroughly.

Teriyaki Pork Roast

Ingredients:

- Pepper to taste
- 4 Tbsp cornstarch mixed with 4 tsp cold water
- 2 Tbsp sugar
- 1 Tbsp white vinegar
- 2 /8 tsp garlic powder
- 4 lb pork loin roast, halved
- 6 Tbsp unsweetened apple juice
- 2 Tbsp reduced-sodium soy sauce
- 1 tsp ground ginger

Instructions:

1. Add apple juice, soy sauce, ginger, pepper, sugar, vinegar and garlic powder into the slow cooker and stir.
2. Place roast in the pot and turn it around in the mixture to coat well.

3. Cover and cook for 8 to 8 hours on low or 4 to 4 hours on high or until roast is cooked through.

4. Remove pork with a slotted spoon and place in a serving bowl. Keep warm.

5. Remove the fat that is floating on the top in the slow cooker.

6. Pour the cooked liquid into a saucepan.

7. Place saucepan over high heat.

8. Add cornstarch mixture and stir constantly until thick.

9. Spoon sauce over the pork and serve.

Slow-Cooker Sausage & Apple Stuffing

Ingredients:

- 2 medium fresh onion, chopped
- 4 oz sweet Italian sausage, discard casing, crumbled
- 1 lb stale, whole grain bread, cubed
- 1 cup low-sodium chicken broth
- 4 Tbsp extra-virgin olive oil
- 2 cup chopped celery
- 2 tsp poultry seasoning or to taste
- Salt to taste
- Pepper to taste
- 2 medium Granny Smith apple, peeled, cored, chopped

Instructions:

1. Place a skillet over medium heat.
2. Add oil and heat.
3. Add celery and onion and sauté until slightly tender.
4. Stir in the sausage, pepper, salt and poultry seasoning and cook until meat is not pink anymore.
5. Turn off the heat and add into the slow cooker.
6. Stir in the bread, broth and apple.
7. Mix until well coated.
8. Cover and cook for 2 hours on high or for 4 hours on low.

Velvety Beef Steak

Ingredients:
- 4 cups thickly sliced onions
- 4 cups green bell pepper strips
- 30 oz low sodium cream of mushroom soup
- 4 lb beef round steak
- 1/2 cup almond flour
- 4 Tbsp olive oil

Instructions:

1. Slice the steak into 10 pieces and coat in the flour.

2. Place nonstick skillet over medium flame and heat the olive oil.

3. Brown the steak all over, then transfer into the slow cooker.

4. Add the bell pepper and onions on top and pour in the soup.

5. Cover and cook for 6 hours on low.

Chili Beef Roast

Ingredients:

- 4 Tbsp chili powder
- 4 Tbsp prepared mustard
- 4 Tbsp Worcestershire sauce
- 4 tsp cider vinegar
- 4 tsp coconut sugar
- 6 potatoes, scrubbed and sliced
- 4 cups sliced onion
- 6 lb beef chuck roast
- 4 Tbsp almond flour
- 4 Tbsp chili sauce

Instructions:

1. In a very large bowl, mix together the flour, chili sauce and powder, Worcestershire sauce, prepared mustard, cider vinegar, and sugar.

2. Toss the beef chuck roast in the mixture, then transfer everything into the slow cooker.

3. Arrange the potatoes on top, then the onions.

4. Cover and cook for 7 hours on low.

Tender Mexican Brisket

Ingredients:
- 4 Tbsp vinegar
- 4 tsp garlic powder
- 1/3 tsp oregano
- 1/3 tsp cinnamon
- 1/2 tsp cloves
- 1/2 tsp pepper
- 1/2 cup water
- 4 Tbsp olive oil
- 6 lb cubed beef brisket
- 4 cups low sodium salsa

Instructions:

1. Place a skillet over medium high flame and heat the olive oil.

2. Brown the beef brisket all over, then transfer into the slow cooker.

3. Add the salsa, vinegar, garlic powder, oregano, cinnamon, cloves, and pepper.

4. Pour in the water.

5. Cover and cook for 7 hours on low.

6. Add more water, if necessary.

Beef With Tangy Horseradish Sauce

Ingredients:

- 4 cups chopped onion
- 10 oz unsalted tomato paste
- 1/2 cup horseradish sauce
- 4 Tbsp olive oil
- 4 lb beef chuck roast
- 1/2 tsp black pepper

Instructions:

1. Place a skillet over medium high flame and heat the olive oil.
2. Brown the beef all over.
3. Transfer into the slow cooker.

4. In a bowl, mix together the black pepper, fresh onion, tomato paste, and horseradish sauce.

5. Pour into the slow cooker and toss the beef to coat.

6. Cover and cook for 25 hours on low.

Sweet Potato And Pork Chops

Ingredients:
- 4 Tbsp olive oil
- 4 sweet potatoes, peeled and cubed
- 4 cups low sodium chicken
- 6 pork loin chops
- 4 cups sliced onions

broth

Instructions:

1. Place a skillet over medium high flame and heat the oil.

2. Brown the pork chops all over.

3. Drain on paper towels.

4. Grease the slow cooker with nonstick cooking spray, then place the sliced onions in the bottom. Put the pork chops over the onions, followed by the sweet potatoes.

5. Add the broth, cover, and cook for 6 hours on low.

North Carolina Pork Roast

Ingredients:
- 1/3 cup cider vinegar
- 1/3 Tbsp hot pepper sauce
- 2 Tbsp coconut sugar
- 1 tsp cayenne
- 4 lb pork shoulder roast
- 1 tsp black pepper

Instructions:

1. Season the pork roast with black pepper, then place into the slow cooker.

2. Add the vinegar into the slow cooker.

3. Cover and cook for 7 hours on low.

4. Take the pork out of the slow cooker and remove the bones.

5. Shred the meat and return into the slow cooker.

6. Strain the liquids from the slow cooker and set aside 2 cup.

7. Stir the sugar, hot pepper sauce, and cayenne into the liquids and pour into the slow cooker.

8. Mix well with the meat.

9. Cover and cook for an additional hour on low.

Cranberry Pork Roast

Ingredients:
- 1/7 cup raw honey or agave nectar
- 1/3 tsp grated orange peel
- Cloves
- Nutmeg
- 2 lb pork loin roast, sliced into 6 pieces
- 1/7 tsp black pepper
- 1/3 lb cranberry sauce with whole cranberries

Instructions:

1. Put the roast into the slow cooker and season with black pepper.

2. In a bowl, mix together the cranberry sauce, honey or agave, orange peel, and a dash of cloves and nutmeg.

3. Mix well, then pour into the slow cooker.

4. Cover and cook for 6 hours on low, or until the meat thermometer shows 2 60 degrees F.

5. Turn off the heat and let it stand for at least 8 minutes before serving.

Pork With Peach And Cherry Salsa

Ingredients:
- 4 tsp canola oil
- 1/2 cup water
- 4 cups frozen unsweetened peach slices, thawed
- 4 cups frozen dark sweet cherries, thawed
- 2 large jalapeno pepper, seeded, minced
- 4 tsp grated peeled ginger root
- 2 tsp balsamic vinegar
- 4 Tbsp Sucanat or xylithol
- 4 tsp chili powder
- 1/2 tsp ground allspice
- 1/3 tsp garlic powder
- 1/3 tsp ground cinnamon
- 1/2 tsp sea salt

- 1/7 tsp cayenne pepper
- 4 lb pork tenderloin, fat removed

Instructions:

1. Coat the slow cooker with nonstick cooking spray.

2. Combine the cinnamon, chili powder, garlic powder, salt, cayenne, and allspice in a bowl.

3. Rub the mixture all over the pork very well.

4. Brown the pork all over in the canola oil in a nonstick skillet over medium high flame.

5. Transfer the meat into the slow cooker.

6. Add the water into the skillet and scrape the browned bits from the bottom.

7. Pour around the pork in the slow cooker.

8. Cover and cook for 2 hours on low or for 2 hour on high, or until the meat thermometer shows 250 degrees F.

9. Drain the liquid from the slow cooker and chop the pork into bite sized pieces.

10. Set aside covered to keep warm.

11. Slice the peaches and dark sweet cherries.

12. Increase slow cooker temperature to high, then place the fruit into it.

13. Add the jalapeno pepper, balsamic vinegar, and Sucanat or xylithol. Stir to combine.

14. Cover and cook for 30 minutes.

15. Turn off the heat and add the ginger root.

16. Stir to combine.

17. Arrange the pork on a platter and spoon the salsa around it.

18. Serve at once.

Cuban Orange Pork

Ingredients:
- 2 lb boneless pork loin roast, fat trimmed
- 1/3 tsp olive oil
- 1/3 Tbsp chopped fresh oregano
- 4 Tbsp minced onion
- 2 tsp cumin seeds
- 1/2 tsp grated orange zest
- 2 large garlic clove, minced
- 2 fresh orange, peeled and segmented
- 1/2 tsp sea salt
- 1/2 tsp freshly ground black pepper

Instructions:

1. Place the orange segments into the slow cooker and gently press to extract some of the juices.

2. Season the pork with salt and pepper.

3. Heat the olive oil in a nonstick skillet over medium high flame, then brown the pork all over.

4. Transfer to a platter and set aside.

5. Set heat to medium and sauté the fresh onion, oregano, cumin seeds, garlic, and orange zest.

6. Cook until fragrant, then press the mixture all over the browned pork.

7. Place the pork into the slow cooker, on top of the oranges.

8. Cover and cook for 6 hours on low or for 4 hours on high, or until the meat

thermometer shows the pork is at 250 degrees F.

9. Throw away the orange wedges. Slice the pork and set on a platter.

10.   Serve 25 minutes after slicing.

Fresh Lemon Beef Goulash

Ingredients:
- 1/2 tsp crushed caraway seeds
- 2 /8 tsp sea salt
- 2 /8 tsp crumbled dried thyme
- 6 oz green beans, trimmed, chopped
- 2 Tbsp minced fresh lemon zest
- Optional: 2 Tbsp zero fat sour cream
- 2 cup halved baby carrots
- 1/3 lb boneless top round roast, visible fat trimmed, cubed
- 2 fresh fresh onion, diced
- 2 Tbsp uncooked quick cooking or instant tapioca
- 1 lb unpeeled red potatoes, scrubbed and cubed
- 1 cup low sodium beef broth
- 1 Tbsp. paprika

- 4 Tbsp unsalted tomato paste
- 2 medium garlic clove, minced
- 1/2 tsp crumbled dried marjoram

Instructions:

1. Place the carrots in a single layer in the slow cooker, followed by the fresh onion, then the beef, and potatoes.
2. Add the tapioca on top. Do not mix.
3. In a bowl, combine the tomato paste, garlic, broth, paprika, marjoram, salt, caraway seeds, and thyme.
4. Pour the mixture all over the beef. Do not mix.
5. Cover and cook for 6 hours on low or for 4 hours on high, or until the beef is cooked through.

6. Add the green beans and fresh lemon zest, then cover and cook for 45 minutes on high.

7. Divide the mixture into individual servings and top with sour cream, if desired.

8. Serve at once.

Tuscan-Style Pork And Beans

Ingredients:

- 1/2 tsp sea salt
- 1/2 tsp freshly ground black pepper
- 4 garlic cloves, minced
- 4 Tbsp minced fresh rosemary
- 1/3 tsp crushed dried fennel seeds
- 1/2 cup dried Great Northern beans, rinsed and drained
- 1/2 cup low sodium chicken broth
- 2 lb boneless pork loin roast, excess fat trimmed
- 2 medium bell pepper, chopped
- 1/3 tsp olive oil

Instructions:

1. Boil water in a saucepan over high flame, then add the beans and bring to a boil.

2. Reduce to a simmer and let simmer for 30 minutes.

3. Drain and rinse thoroughly.

4. Transfer the beans into the slow cooker.

5. Add the broth and bell pepper into the slow cooker.

6. Place a nonstick skillet over medium high flame and heat the olive oil.

7. Brown the pork all over, then transfer to a platter and season with the salt and pepper.

8. Set aside.

9. Combine the garlic, rosemary, and crushed fennel seeds.

10. Rub the mixture all over one side of the pork.

11. Place the pork, unseasoned side down, in the slow cooker, on top of the beans.

12. Cover and cook for 25 hours on low or for 6-6 ½ hours on high, or until the pork and beans are tender.

13. Take the pork out of the slow cooker and slice.

14. Transfer the beans to a serving bowl and place the sliced pork on top. Serve warm.

Beef Picadillo

Ingredients:

- 1 tsp ground cumin
- 1 tsp garlic powder
- 1 tsp ground nutmeg
- 1/3 tsp ground cinnamon
- 1 tsp crumbled dried thyme
- 1/2 tsp ground allspice
- 1/2 tsp sea salt
- 1/2 tsp freshly ground black pepper
- 25 oz frozen brown rice
- 1/2 cup dry roasted slivered almonds
- 7 oz lean ground beef
- 1/2 cup golden or dark raisins
- 2 4.6 oz unsalted diced tomatoes, undrained
- 2 bay leaf

- 2 fresh onion, diced
- 2 tsp Sucanat
- 2 fresh jalapeno or Serrano pepper, minced

Instructions:

1. Coat the slow cooker with nonstick cooking spray.

2. Brown the beef in a nonstick skillet over medium high flame, then transfer to the slow cooker.

3. Add the bay leaves, tomatoes with their juices, raisins, fresh onion, sugar, cinnamon, pepper, cumin, nutmeg, thyme, allspice, and garlic powder into the slow cooker.

4. Cover and cook for 4 hours on high or for 6 hours on low.

5. Prepare the rice based on manufacturer's instructions.

6. Divide into separate servings.

7. Remove the bay leaves from the slow cooker.

8. Add the salt, pepper, and almonds.

9. Divide the picadillo beef into equal portions on top of the rice. Serve warm.

Pork And Potato Casserole

Ingredients:
- 2 tsp crumbled dried thyme
- 2 tsp caraway seeds
- 1/2 tsp sea salt
- 1/7 tsp freshly ground black pepper
- 4 Tbsp cornstarch
- 1/3 cup low sodium beef broth
- 1/2 cup low sodium chicken broth
- 2 red bell pepper, sliced into rings
- 4 tsp olive oil, divided
- 6 boneless pork chops, 4 oz each, visible fat trimmed
- 2 large fresh onion, sliced
- 2 large garlic clove, minced
- 4 lb red potatoes, peeled and sliced

Instructions:

1. Coat the slow cooker with nonstick cooking spray and set aside.

2. Heat half of the olive oil over medium high flame in a skillet, then brown the pork all over.

3. Transfer to a plate and set aside.

4. Heat the remaining oil in the skillet, then reduce the heat and sauté the onions until golden.

5. Turn off the heat and set aside.

6. Place half of the sliced potatoes into the slow cooker, then add half the onions on top.

7. Season with caraway seeds, salt, pepper, thyme, and half of the garlic.

8. Place the browned pork on top. Repeat the potato, fresh onion, and garlic layers.

9. Pour the beef broth into the skillet and simmer over medium flame.

10. Combine the chicken broth and cornstarch in a bowl, mixing well.

11. Stir the mixture into the skillet with the beef broth and simmer until thickened.

12. Pour the mixture into the slow cooker.

13. Cover the slow cooker and cook for 6 hours on low, or until the meat thermometer shows the pork is at 250 degrees F.

14. Top the casserole with the bell pepper rings.

15. Cover and cook for 25 minutes. Serve warm.

Basil Pork Chops With Grape Tomatoes

Ingredients:
- 4 tsp olive oil
- 2 cups grape tomatoes, halved
- 1 cups white wine or low sodium chicken broth
- 4 Tbsp chopped fresh basil
- 4 garlic cloves, minced
- 6 lean pork rib chops, 6 oz each, bone in, fat removed
- 1/2 tsp sea salt
- 1/2 tsp freshly ground black pepper

Instructions:

1. Season the pork with the garlic, salt and pepper.

2. Heat the oil over medium high flame in a skillet, then brown the pork all over.

3. Transfer to the slow cooker.

4. Arrange the pork in a single layer, overlapping the ends if needed.

5. Add the wine or broth into the skillet, then bring to a boil.

6. Scrape the bottom to loosen the browned bits.

7. Continue to boil for 5 minute or until the liquid is reduced to half.

8. Pour the liquid into the slow cooker.

9. Place the halved grape tomatoes on top of the pork.

10. Cover and cook on low for 4 hours and 45 minutes, or on high for 2 hours, or until the meat thermometer shows the pork is at 250 degrees F.

11. Place the pork onto a serving platter.

12. Take the tomatoes out of the slow cooker using a slotted spoon and place them around the pork.

13. Transfer the cooking liquid to a skillet and boil over high heat for 5 minutes until thickened.

14. Pour all over the dish. Top with fresh basil, then serve.

Chinese Ginger And Beef

Ingredients:
- 2 fresh onion chopped
- 1/3 cup low sodium beef broth
- 2 Tbsp soy sauce
- 2 Tbsp grated fresh ginger
- 2 oz frozen peas
- 1 Tbsp corn flour
- 4 Tbsp water
- sea salt
- Pepper
- 1/3 lb round steak, cubed
- 2 carrots, peeled and sliced
- 2 garlic clove, crushed
- 1 red bell pepper, seeded and sliced

Instructions:

1. Place the carrots, bell pepper, and garlic in the slow cooker.

2. Add the beef on top and scatter the onion.

3. Add the soy sauce, ginger, and low sodium beef broth, then season with a dash each of sea salt and pepper.

4. Cover and cook for 6 hours on low or for 4 hours on high.

5. Combine the corn flour and water in a bowl then add into the slow cooker.

6. Stir to combine, then add the peas.

7. Cover and cook for an additional 25 minutes or until beef and peas are cooked through. Serve hot.

Lean Meatloaf

Ingredients:
- 2 fresh egg
- 1/2 sweet fresh onion, minced
- 1/2 cup whole rolled oats
- 1 fresh bell pepper, seeded and minced
- 1 tsp sea salt
- 1/2 tsp cracked black pepper
- 1 lb extra lean ground turkey
- 1 lb extra lean ground beef
- 1/3 Tbsp Worcestershire sauce, organic
- 1 lb baby carrots
- 1/2 cup low sugar barbecue sauce or ketchup

Instructions:

1. Spread the carrots in the slow cooker in an even layer.

2. Whisk the egg in a bowl and mix in the Worcestershire sauce, fresh onion, oats, bell pepper, and half of the barbecue sauce or ketchup.

3. Mix in the beef and turkey, then season with sea salt and pepper.

4. Mix with hands, but do not over mix to avoid a dry loaf.

5. Pack the meat mixture into the slow cooker on top of the carrots, then cover and cook for 4 hours on low, or until the meat loaf is completely cooked.

6. Increase heat to high, then pour the remaining barbecue sauce or ketchup on top.

7. Cook for an additional 25 minutes, then serve.

Raspberry & Coconut Cake

Ingredients:

- 4 large fresh eggs
- 1 cup melted coconut oil
- ¾ cup of coconut milk
- 2 cup raspberries, fresh or frozen
- 1 cup sugarless dark chocolate chips
- 2 cups ground almonds
- 2 cup shredded coconut
- ¾ cup sweetener, Swerve
- 2 teaspoon baking soda
- 1/2 teaspoon salt

Directions:

1. Butter the crockpot.
2. In a bowl, mix the dry ingredients.
3. Beat in the fresh eggs, melted coconut oil, and coconut milk.

4. Mix in the raspberries plus chocolate chips.
5. Combine the cocoa, almonds, and salt in a bowl.
6. Pour the batter into the buttered crockpot.
7. Cover the crockpot with a paper towel to absorb the water.
8. Cover, cook on low for 4 hours. Let the cake cool in the pot.

Chocolate Cheesecake

Ingredients:

- 2 cup powder sweetener of your choice, Swerve
- 2 teaspoon vanilla extract
- 1 cup sugarless dark chocolate chips
- 4 cups cream cheese
- Pinch of salt
- 4 fresh eggs

Directions:

1. Whisk the cream cheese, sweetener, and salt in a bowl.
2. Add the eggs one at a time. Combine thoroughly.
3. Spread the cheesecake in a cake pan, which fits in the crockpot you are using.
4. Dissolved the chocolate chips in a fresh pot and pour over the batter.
5. Using a knife, swirl the chocolate through the batter.
6. Put 2 cups of water inside the crockpot and set the cake pan inside.
7. Cover it with a paper towel to absorb the water, then cook on high for 2.6 hours.
8. Remove from the crockpot and let it cool in the pan for 2 hour. Refrigerate.

Crème Brule

Ingredients:
- 2 cups double cream
- 2 Bourbon vanilla pod, scraped
- Pinch of salt
- 6 large egg yolks
- 6 Tablespoons sweetener, Erythritol

Directions:
1. In a bowl, beat the eggs and sweetener together.
2. Add the cream and vanilla. Whisk together.
3. Put it in one big dish.
4. Set it in the crockpot and pour hot water around- so the water reaches halfway up the dish.
5. Cover, cook on high for 2 hours.
6. Take the dishes out, let them cool.
7. Refrigerate for 6-8 hours.

Peanut Butter & Chocolate Cake

Ingredients:
- 2 teaspoon baking powder
- 1/2 teaspoon salt
- ¾ cup peanut butter, melted
- 4 large fresh eggs
- 2 teaspoon vanilla extract
- 1 cup of water
- 4 Tablespoons sugarless dark chocolate, melted
- 2 Tablespoon butter for greasing the crockpot
- 2 cups almond flour
- ¾ cup sweetener of your choice
- 1/2 cup coconut flakes
- 1/2 cup whey protein powder

Directions:

1. Grease the crockpot well.
2. In a bowl, mix the dry ingredients.
3. Stir in the wet ingredients one at a time.
4. Spread about 1/2 of batter in the crockpot, add half the chocolate.
5. Swirl with a fork.
6. Top up with the remaining batter and chocolate.
7. Swirl again.
8. Cook on low for 4 hours.
9. Switch off.
10. Let it sit covered for 45 minutes.

Keto Coconut Hot Chocolate

Ingredients:

- 2 tsp vanilla extract
- 1/2 cup cocoa powder
- 4 ounces dark chocolate, roughly chopped
- 1 tsp cinnamon
- Few drops of stevia to taste
- 6 cups full-fat coconut milk
- 2 cups heavy cream

Directions:

1. Add the coconut milk, cream, vanilla extract, cocoa powder, chocolate, cinnamon, and stevia to the crockpot and stir to combine.

2. Cook for 4 hours, high, whisking every 46 minutes.
3. Taste the hot chocolate and if you prefer more sweetness, add a few more drops of stevia.

Ambrosia

Ingredients:

- 4 ounces dark chocolate roughly chopped
- 1/2 cup pumpkin seeds
- 2 ounces salted butter
- 2 tsp cinnamon
- 2 cups heavy cream
- 2 cups full-fat Greek yogurt
- 2 cup fresh berries – strawberries and raspberries are best
- 2 cup unsweetened shredded coconut
- ¾ cup slivered almonds

150

Directions:
1. Place the shredded coconut, slivered almonds, dark chocolate, pumpkin seeds, butter, and cinnamon into the crockpot.
2. Cook for 4 hours, high, stirring every 46 minutes to combine the chocolate and butter as it melts.
3. Remove the mixture from the crockpot, place in a bowl, and leave to cool.
4. In a large bowl, whip the cream until softly whipped.
5. Stir the yogurt through the cream.
6. Slice the strawberries into pieces, then put it to the cream mixture, along with the other berries you are using, fold through.
7. Sprinkle the cooled coconut mixture over the cream mixture.

Dark Chocolate And Peppermint Pots

Ingredients:

- 4 egg yolks, lightly beaten with a fork
- Few drops of stevia
- Few drops of peppermint essence to taste
- 4 cups heavy cream
- 4 ounces dark chocolate, melted in the microwave

Directions:

1. Mix the beaten egg yolks, cream, stevia, melted chocolate, and peppermint essence in a medium-sized bowl.
2. Prepare the pots by greasing 6 ramekins with butter.

3. Pour the chocolate mixture into the pots evenly.
4. Put the pots inside the slow cooker and put hot water below halfway up.
5. Cook for 2 hours, high.
6. Take the pots out of the slow cooker and leave to cool and set.
7. Serve with a fresh mint leaf and whipped cream.

Creamy Vanilla Custard

Ingredients:
- 2 tsp vanilla extract
- Few drops of stevia
- 4 cups full-fat cream
- 4 egg yolks, lightly beaten

Directions:
1. Mix the cream, egg yolks, vanilla extract, and stevia in a medium-sized bowl.
2. Pour the mixture into a heat-proof dish.
3. Place the dish into the slow cooker.
4. Put hot water into the pot, around the dish, halfway up.
5. Set the temperature to high.
6. Cook for 4 hours. Serve hot or cold!

Coconut, Chocolate, And Almond Truffle Bake

Ingredients:

- 2 tsp vanilla extract
- 2 cup heavy cream
- A few extra squares of dark chocolate, grated
- 1/2 cup toasted almonds, chopped
- 4 ounces butter, melted
- 4 ounces dark chocolate, melted
- 2 cup ground almonds
- 2 cup desiccated coconut
- 4 tbsp unsweetened cocoa powder

Directions:

1. In a large bowl, mix the melted butter, chocolate, ground almonds, coconut, cocoa powder, and vanilla extract.

2. Roll the mixture into balls.
3. Grease a heat-proof dish.
4. Place the balls into the dish—Cook for 4 hours, low setting.
5. Leave the truffle dish to cool until warm.
6. Mix the cream until soft peak. Spread the cream over the truffle dish and sprinkle the grated chocolate and chopped toasted almonds over the top. Serve immediately!

Peanut Butter, Chocolate, And Pecan Cupcakes

Ingredients:

- 6 ounces dark chocolate
- 2 tbsp coconut oil
- 2 fresh eggs, lightly beaten
- 2 cup ground almonds
- 2 tsp baking powder
- 2 tsp cinnamon
- 25 pecan nuts, toasted and finely chopped
- 2 4 paper cupcake cases
- 2 cup smooth peanut butter
- 2 ounces butter
- 2 tsp vanilla extract

Directions:

1. Dissolve the dark chocolate plus coconut oil in the microwave, stir to combine, and set aside.
2. Place the peanut butter and butter into a medium-sized bowl, microwave for 45 seconds at a time until the butter has just melted.
3. Mix the peanut butter plus butter until combined and smooth.
4. Stir the vanilla extract into the peanut butter mixture.
5. Mix the ground almonds, fresh eggs, baking powder, and cinnamon in a fresh bowl.
6. Pour the melted chocolate and coconut oil evenly into the 2 4 paper cases.
7. Spoon half of the almond/egg mixture evenly into the cases, on top of the chocolate and press down slightly.

8. Spoon the peanut butter mixture into the cases, on top of the almond/egg mixture.
9. Spoon the remaining almond/egg mixture into the cases.
10. Put the pecans on top of each cupcake.
11. Put the filled cases into the slow cooker—Cook for 4 hours, high setting.

Vanilla And Strawberry Cheesecake

Ingredients:

- 2 tsp cinnamon
- Filling:
- 2 cups cream cheese
- 2 fresh eggs, lightly beaten
- 2 cup sour cream
- 2 tsp vanilla extract
- 8 large strawberries, chopped
- Base:
- 2 ounces butter, melted
- 2 cup ground hazelnuts
- 1 cup desiccated coconut
- 2 tsp vanilla extract

Directions:
1. Mix the melted butter, hazelnuts, coconut, vanilla, and cinnamon in a medium-sized bowl.
2. Press the base into a greased heat-proof dish.
3. Mix the cream cheese, fresh eggs, sour cream, and vanilla extract, beat with electric egg beaters in a large bowl until thick and combined.
4. the strawberries through the cream cheese mixture.
5. Put the cream cheese batter into the dish, on top of the base, spread out until smooth.
6. Put it in the slow cooker and put hot water around the dish until halfway up.
7. Cook for 6 hours, low setting until just set but slightly wobbly.
8. Chill before serving.

Coffee Creams With Toasted Seed Crumble Topping

Ingredients:

- 4 tbsp strong espresso coffee
- 1 cup mixed seeds – sesame seeds, pumpkin seeds, chia seeds, sunflower seeds,
- 2 tsp cinnamon
- 2 cups heavy cream
- 4 egg yolks, lightly beaten
- 2 tsp vanilla extract

2 tbsp coconut oil

Directions:

1. Heat-up the coconut oil in a fresh frypan until melted.
2. Add the mixed seeds, cinnamon, and a pinch of salt, toss in the oil and heat

until toasted and golden, place into a fresh bowl and set aside.
3. Mix the cream, egg yolks, vanilla, and coffee in a medium-sized bowl.
4. Pour the cream/coffee mixture into the ramekins.
5. Place the ramekins into the slow cooker.
6. Put hot water inside until halfway.
7. Cook on low setting for 4 hours.
8. Remove, then leave to cool slightly on the bench.
9. Sprinkle the seed mixture over the top of each custard before serving.

Fresh Lemon Cheesecake

Ingredients:

- 2 tsp cinnamon
- 2 cups cream cheese
- 2 cup sour cream
- 2 fresh eggs, lightly beaten
- 2 fresh lemon
- Few drops of stevia
- 2 cup heavy cream
- 2 ounces butter, melted
- 2 cup pecans, finely ground in the food processor

Directions:

1. Mix the melted butter, ground pecans, and cinnamon until it forms a wet, sand-like texture.

2. Press the butter/pecan mixture into a greased, heat-proof dish and set aside.
3. Place the cream cheese, fresh eggs, sour cream, stevia, zest, and juice of one fresh lemon into a large bowl, beat with electric egg beaters until combined and smooth.
4. Put the cream cheese batter into the dish, on top of the base.
5. Place the dish inside the slow cooker, then put warm water in halfway up.
6. Cook within 6 hours, low setting.
7. Set the cheesecake on the bench to cool and set.
8. Whip the cream until soft peak, and spread over the cheesecake before serving.

Apple, Avocado And Mango Bowls

Ingredients:

- 2 apple, cored and cubed
- tablespoons brown sugar
- 2 cup heavy cream
- 2 tablespoon fresh lemon juice
- 2 cup avocado, peeled, pitted and cubed
- 2 cup mango, peeled and cubed

Directions:

1. In your slow cooker, combine the avocado with the mango and the other ingredients, toss gently, put the lid on and cook on Low for 2 hours.
2. Divide the mix into bowls and serve.

Ricotta Cream

Ingredients:

- and 1 teaspoons gelatin
- 2 teaspoon vanilla extract
- 2 teaspoon espresso powder
- 2 teaspoon sugar
- 2 cup whipping cream
- 1 cup hot coffee
- cups ricotta cheese

Directions:

1. In a bowl, mix coffee with gelatin, stir well and leave aside until coffee is cold.
2. In your slow cooker, mix espresso, sugar, vanilla extract and ricotta and stir.

3. Add coffee mix and whipping cream, cover, cook on Low for 2 hour.
4. Divide into dessert bowls and keep in the fridge for 2 hours before serving.

Tomato Jam

Ingredients

- tablespoons red wine vinegar
- tablespoons sugar
- 1 pound tomatoes, chopped
- 2 green apple, grated

Directions:

1. In your slow cooker, mix the tomatoes with the apple with the other ingredients, put the lid on and cook on Low for 4 hours.
2. Whisk the jam well, blend a bit using an immersion blender, divide into bowls and serve cold.

Green Tea Pudding

Ingredients:

- tablespoons green tea powder
- teaspoons lime zest, grated
- 2 tablespoon sugar
- 1 cup coconut milk
- 2 and 1 cup avocado, pitted and peeled

Directions:

1. In your slow cooker, mix coconut milk with avocado, tea powder, lime zest and sugar, stir, cover and cook on Low for 2 hour.
2. Divide into cups and serve cold.

Sweet Fresh Lemon Mix

Ingredients:

- Sugar to the taste
- lemons, peeled and roughly chopped
- cups heavy cream

Directions:

1. In your slow cooker, mix cream with sugar and lemons, stir, cover and cook on Low for 2 hour.
2. Divide into glasses and serve very cold.

Coconut Jam

Ingredients:

- 2 cup coconut cream
- 1 cup heavy cream
- tablespoons sugar
- 2 tablespoon fresh lemon juice
- 1 cup coconut flesh, shredded

Directions:

1. In your slow cooker, mix the coconut cream with the fresh lemon juice, add other ingredients, whisk, put the lid on and cook on Low for 2 hours.
2. Whisk well, divide into bowls and serve cold.

Banana Bread

Ingredients:

- bananas, mashed
- 2 teaspoon baking powder
- 2 and 1 cups flour
- 1 teaspoons baking soda
- 1/2 cup milk
- 2 and 1 teaspoons cream of tartar
- Cooking spray
- ¾ cup sugar
- 1/2 cup butter, soft
- 2 teaspoon vanilla extract
- 2 fresh egg

Directions:

1. In a bowl, combine milk with cream of tartar and stir well.
2. Add sugar, butter, egg, vanilla and bananas and stir everything. In another bowl, mix flour with salt, baking powd
3. er and soda.
4. Combine the 2 mixtures and stir them well.
5. Grease your slow cooker with cooking spray, add bread `batter, cover, and cook on High for 4 hours.
6. Leave the bread to cool down, slice and serve it.

Bread And Berries Pudding

Ingredients:

- tablespoons white sugar
- 2 cup almond milk
- 1/2 cup heavy cream - fresh eggs, whisked
- 2 tablespoon fresh lemon zest, grated
- 1/2 teaspoon vanilla extract
- cups white bread, cubed
- 2 cup blackberries
- tablespoons butter, melted

Directions:

1. In your slow cooker, mix the bread with the berries, butter and the other ingredients, toss gently, put the lid on and cook on Low for 4 hours.

2. Divide pudding between dessert plates and serve.

Candied Lemon

Ingredients:

- cups white sugar
- cups water
- lemons, peeled and cut into medium segments

Directions:

1. In your slow cooker, mix lemons with sugar and water, cover, cook on Low for 4 hours, transfer them to bowls and serve cold.

Tapioca And Chia Pudding

Ingredients:
- fresh eggs, whisked
- 1 teaspoon vanilla extract
- tablespoons sugar
- 1 tablespoon fresh lemon zest, grated
- 2 cup almond milk
- 1/2 cup tapioca pearls
- tablespoons chia seeds

Directions:
3. In your slow cooker, mix the tapioca pearls with the milk, put the lid on and cook on Low for 4 hours.
4. Divide the pudding into bowls and serve cold.

Lightning Source UK Ltd.
Milton Keynes UK
UKHW052225061022
410070UK00016B/134